Copyright 2023

All right reserved.No part of this book should be reproduced without express permission of the author.

Reproduction of all or any part of this book is punishable unders relevant law.

1

Table of Contents

Crohn's disease is a type of inflammatory bowel disease (IBD). It causes swelling of the tissues (inflammation) in your digestive tract, which can lead to abdominal pain, severe diarrhea, fatigue, weight loss and malnutrition.

Inflammation caused by Crohn's disease can involve different areas of the digestive tract in different people, most commonly the small intestine. This inflammation often spreads into the deeper layers of the bowel.

Crohn's disease can be both painful and debilitating, and sometimes may lead to life-threatening complications.

There's no known cure for Crohn's disease, but therapies can greatly reduce its signs and symptoms and even bring about long-term remission and healing of inflammation. With treatment, many people with Crohn's disease are able to function well.

BREAKFAST

1. Vegan Burrito

Prep Time: 25 Minutes

Cook Time: 10 Minutes

Servings: 4-6

Ingredients

Creamy Siracha Sauce:

- 1/4 cup siracha sauce
- 2 tablespoons Califia Unsweetened Almondmilk

Tofu Scramble:

- 1 14oz package extra firm tofu
- 1 tablespoon olive or avocado oil
- 1–2 teaspoons garlic, minced
- 1 small yellow onion, diced
- 1/2 – 1 teaspoon kosher salt
- 1/4 teaspoon ground black pepper
- 1–2 teaspoons ground turmeric

Other Burrito Ingredients:

- 1 15oz can black beans, drained
- 1 avocado, sliced
- 1 cup fresh spinach
- 4 large burrito tortillas (or about 6–8 regular sized ones)

Instructions

Creamy Siracha Sauce

1. Combine Creamy Siracha Sauce Ingredients in small bow, mix well and set aside.

Tofu Scramble

2. Place tofu on plate or pan.
3. Use fork to break it up into chunks (you will break it up even more in the pan so it doesn't have to be perfect) and set aside.
4. Bring large cast iron skillet to medium high heat.
5. Add olive oil and swirl to coat the pan.
6. Add garlic and let cook until fragrant, about 1 minute.
7. Add onion and allow to cook down, about 1-2 minutes.
8. Turn heat down to medium/medium-low.

9. Add tofu and move around the pan breaking up any larger tofu chunks until it looks like scrambled eggs.

10. Add salt, pepper and turmeric; mix well to combine.

11. Taste and add any additional seasoning, as desired.

Make Breakfast Burrito

1. Take tortilla and place Creamy Siracha Sauce, tofu scramble, back beans, spinach and avocado in the center.

2. Fold in both sides, take the end of the tortilla closest to you and wrap over the ingredients (away from you) tucking in any stray ingredients. Continue rolling away from you until you have a burrito!

3. Continue in the same fashion until all your burritos are made.

Prep Time: 10 Minutes

Cook Time: 15 Minutes

Servings: 4

Ingredients

- 6oz smoked chorizo sausage, cut into thick slices and then quarter each slice.
- 2 yams or sweet potatoes (I used a yam and a purple sweet potato); cubed
- pinch of salt
- 1 Tablespoon olive oil
- 1 Tablespoons of bacon grease or ghee
- Serving suggestions:
- paleo tortillas
- 2 fried eggs
- avocado
- micro-greens

Instructions

1. Heat large skillet to medium heat.

2. Add olive oil and sweet potatoes.

3. Stir potatoes on and off until they are firm, but you can still pierce with a fork (approx. 7-8 minutes).

4. Add chorizo and stir until it is thoroughly heat.

5. Add bacon grease or ghee, stir and let sit for 2-3 minutes, reducing heat to medium-low.

6. Serve immediately either in a paleo taco, with eggs or just serve it alone!

Prep Time: 10 Minutes

Cook Time: 10 Minutes

Servings: 2

Ingredients

- 1 small French baguette (cut in half both lengthwise and width-wise)
- 4 eggs
- 4 slices of bacon
- 1 cup of spinach/arugula mix
- 1 cup of Hollandaise Sauce
- salt and pepper to taste

Instructions

1. Hollandaise Sauce should be prepared ahead of time and sitting in a bowl, placed over a large stew pot with about an inch of hot water at the bottom to keep the sauce warm. Add a Tablespoon of warm water and whisk into the sauce to revive it after it sits for a bit.

2. Cut long bacon strips in half and fry until reached your desired crispiness.

3. Prepare French Baguette on plate and have spinach/arugula mix prepped and ready to use.

4. Have Hollandaise sauce ready to go.

5. In shallow sauce pan, fill about 2 -3 inches of water and bring to almost a boil (it is best right when the water starts to bubble of the bottom of the pan).

6. Crack egg into a small glass liquid measuring cup and slowly, very slowly, pour into water.

7. Let cook about 2-3 minutes, depending upon how cooked you want your eggs.

8. While the egg cooks, take a piece of the baguette, place on plate, top with bacon, and then spinach/arugula.

9. Remove eggs with slotted spoon and place on top of the spinach/arugula.

10. Pour Hollandaise sauce over everything and season with salt and pepper.

11. Serve immediately.

Prep Time: 10 Minutes

Cook Time: 10 Minutes

Servings: 1

Ingredients

- 3 egg whites
- 2 Tablespoons chopped spinach
- 1.3 oz soft goat cheese
- Approx. 1/2 cup cherry tomatoes (the more colorful the better) – washed and cut in half lengthwise
- salt to taste and ground black pepper

Instructions

1. In small bowl, add egg whites and spinach; mix.
2. Add egg white mixture to omelette pan on medium heat.
3. Turn on broiler on high and place tomatoes on cookie sheet lined with foil – don't put in oven yet.
4. Use spatula to gently slide under the omelette on all sides as it starts to cook.

5. Continue working the spatula under the omelette, ensuring it isn't sticking.

6. Once omelette is fully cooked on the side that is down, carefully use a spatula (or two) to quickly flip it over.

7. Put tomatoes in the oven for approx. 3 minutes or until tomatoes are starting to sizzle.

8. Using your (clean) hands, place chunks of goat cheese all over one half of the omelette.

9. Fold other side of omelette over the other and let goat cheese melt.

10. Take out tomatoes.

11. Plate omelette and sprinkle with kosher salt and ground black pepper.

12. Serve tomatoes on top of omelette.

Prep Time: 30 Minutes

Cook Time: 3hrs 30 Minutes

Servings: 8-10

Ingredients

- 1 5-6 pound first-cut (or flat-cut) beef brisket, trimmed so a thin layer of fat remains in some spots (do not over trim!)
- 1½ tablespoons salt
- 1 teaspoon ground black pepper
- 2 tablespoons all-purpose flour (okay to substitute matzo cake meal for Passover)
- 3 tablespoons vegetable oil
- 8 medium yellow onions, peeled and sliced ½-inch thick
- 3 tablespoons tomato paste
- 3 cloves garlic, roughly chopped
- 6 carrots, peeled and sliced into large chunks on a diagonal
- Handful fresh chopped parsley, for garnish (optional)

Instructions

1. Set an oven rack in the middle position and preheat the oven to 350°F.

2. Season the brisket on both sides with the salt and pepper. Lightly dust the brisket with the flour, then shake and turn to coat evenly. Heat the oil over medium-high heat in a heavy flameproof roasting pan or ovenproof enameled cast-iron pot just large enough to hold the brisket and carrots snugly. Add the brisket to the pan and sear on both sides until crusty brown areas appear on the surface, 5 to 7 minutes per side.

3. Transfer the brisket to a platter, then add the onions to the pot and stir constantly with a wooden spoon, scraping up any browned bits stuck to the bottom of the pot. Cook until the onions are softened and golden brown, about 15 minutes. (If browned bits stick to the bottom of the pan and start to burn, add a few tablespoons of water and scrape with a wooden spoon to release them.)

4. Turn off the heat and place the brisket, fatty side up, and any accumulated juices on top of the onions. Spread the tomato paste evenly over the brisket, then scatter the garlic and carrots around the edges of the pot. Cover the pot very tightly with aluminum foil

(preferably heavy-duty or two layers) or a lid, then transfer to the oven and cook for 1½ hours.

5. Transfer the brisket to a cutting board and, using an electric or very sharp knife, slice the meat across the grain into approximately ⅛ - ¼-inch-thick slices. Return the slices to the pot, overlapping them at an angle so that you can see a bit of the top edge of each slice. The end result should resemble the original unsliced brisket leaning slightly backward. Cover the pot tightly and return to the oven.

6. Lower the heat to 325°F and cook the brisket until it is fork-tender, 1¾ to 2½ hours, or longer if necessary. The brisket is ready to serve with its juices, but it is even better the second day. (Note: If the sauce seems greasy, transfer the meat and vegetables to a platter and cover with foil to keep warm. Pour the sauce into a bowl and let sit until the fat rises to the top. Using a small ladle, spoon out the fat. Pour the skimmed gravy back over the meat.)

7. Make-Ahead/Freezer-Friendly Instructions: The brisket can be made up to 3 days ahead of time and refrigerated. Reheat the brisket in a 300°F oven until hot, about 45 minutes. The brisket also freezes well

for up to 2 months; defrost in the refrigerator 2 days
ahead of time.

Prep Time: 10 Minutes

Cook Time: 30 Minutes

Servings: 6

Ingredients

- 2 tablespoons vegetable oil
- 6 bratwurst
- 2 medium yellow onions, thinly sliced
- ½ teaspoon salt
- 1 (12 oz) bottle lager beer

For Serving (Optional):

- 6 hoagie rolls or hot dog buns
- Coarse grain mustard
- Warm sauerkraut

Instructions

1. In a large (12-inch) cast iron skillet or nonstick pan with a tight-fitting lid, heat the oil over medium-high heat. Add the bratwurst and sear until nicely

browned, 2 to 3 minutes per side. Using tongs, transfer the sausage to a plate; set aside. Add the onions and salt to the skillet and cook, stirring frequently, until the onions are softened and golden brown, about 5 minutes (do not burn; reduce the heat if necessary).

2. Place the bratwurst back in the pan on top of the onions, add the beer, and bring to a boil. Reduce the heat to low, cover with the lid, and simmer for 10 minutes (at this point the sausages will be partially cooked through). Remove the cover, increase the heat to medium, and continue cooking until the bratwurst are cooked through and the beer is reduced by about three quarters, 10 to 12 minutes more. Serve the bratwurst and onions on rolls with mustard and sauerkraut, if desired.

3. I use Johnsonville Original Brats; avoid any brats already flavored with beer, as the finished dish will taste too bitter. Also be sure to purchase fresh (not cooked) sausages.

4. Lager is a family of beers that includes bright lagers, amber lagers, dark lagers, Oktoberfests, and pilsners. I use Sam Adams Oktoberfest, but Budweiser, Bud

Light, Coors Light, and Miller Lite are all good options. No need to use anything fancy!

Prep Time: 25 Minutes

Cook Time: 40 Minutes

Servings: 6-8

Ingredients

- 2 cups old-fashioned rolled oats (not instant)
- ⅔ cup packed dark brown sugar
- 1 cup chopped pecans, divided
- 1 teaspoon baking powder
- 2 teaspoons ground cinnamon
- ¼ teaspoon ground nutmeg
- ½ teaspoon salt
- 2 large eggs
- 1⅓ cups milk
- 1 teaspoon vanilla extract
- 3 tablespoons unsalted butter, melted, plus more for greasing the dish
- 2½ cups blueberries, divided
- Lightly sweetened Greek yogurt, for serving (optional)

Instructions

1. Preheat the oven to 350°F and set an oven rack in the middle position. Grease an 8-inch or 2-quart baking dish with butter.

2. In a medium bowl, combine the oats, brown sugar, ¼ cup of the nuts, baking powder, cinnamon, nutmeg, and salt. Mix well.

3. In another bowl, break up the eggs with a whisk; then whisk in the milk and vanilla until well combined. Add the milk mixture to the oat mixture, along with the melted butter.

4. Scatter 2 cups of the blueberries evenly over the bottom of the prepared baking dish. Pour the oatmeal mixture over top and spread evenly. Sprinkle the remaining ¾ cup nuts and ½ cup blueberries on top. Bake for 45 to 55 minutes, until the pecans on top are a rich brown color and the oats are set. Let cool for at least 5 minutes, then serve warm or at room temperature with Greek yogurt, if desired.

5. Freezer-Friendly Instructions: This dish can be frozen after baking, tightly covered, for up to 3 months. When you're ready to serve it, defrost in the refrigerator for 24 hours then reheat it, covered with foil, in a 325°F oven until hot.

Prep Time: 25 Minutes

Cook Time: 40 Minutes

Servings: 8

Ingredients

- 1¼ cups all-purpose flour, spooned into measuring cup and leveled-off
- ¼ cup natural unsweetened cocoa powder,
- 1 teaspoon baking soda
- 1 teaspoon salt
- 1 stick (½ cup) unsalted butter, at room temperature
- 1 cup sugar
- 2 large eggs
- 1 cup mashed very ripe bananas, from 2-3 brown bananas
- ½ cup sour cream
- 1 teaspoon vanilla
- ½ cup semi-sweet chocolate chips

Instructions

1. Preheat the oven to 350° F. Grease a 9 x 5 x 3-inch loaf pan with non-stick cooking spray.

2. In a medium bowl, combine the flour, cocoa powder, baking soda and salt. Whisk until there are no more lumps in the cocoa powder and the mixture is well combined. Set aside.

3. In a large bowl or electric mixer fitted with the paddle attachment or beaters, beat the butter and sugar until light and fluffy, 2 to 3 minutes. Add the eggs one at a time, incorporating well after each addition. Add the dry ingredients and beat gently until just combined. Add the bananas, sour cream and vanilla and mix on low speed to combine. Fold in the chocolate chips. Do not overmix.

4. Pour the batter into the prepared loaf pan and spread evenly with a spatula. Bake until a toothpick inserted into the center comes out with a few moist crumbs attached, about 1 hour and 10 minutes. Let the loaf rest in the pan for about 10 minutes, run a blunt knife around the edges to loosen, then turn it out onto a rack to cool completely.

5. There are two types of unsweetened cocoa powder: natural (such as Hershey's) and Dutch-processed. Dutch-processed will not work in this recipe.

6. Freezer-Friendly Instructions: The bread can be frozen for up to 3 months. After it is completely cooled, wrap it securely in aluminum foil, freezer wrap or place in a freezer bag. Thaw overnight in the refrigerator before serving.

Prep Time: 55 Minutes

Cook Time: 30 Minutes

Servings: 4

Ingredients

- 2 racks baby back pork ribs (4-5 pounds), membrane removed (see note below)
- 1 cup hoisin sauce, best quality such as Kikkoman
- ½ cup chili sauce (preferably Heinz)
- 2½ tablespoons dry Sherry
- 2 tablespoons honey
- 2 tablespoons soy sauce (use gluten-free if needed)
- 1½ tablespoons seasoned rice vinegar
- ½ teaspoon Asian/toasted sesame oil
- 4 cloves garlic, minced
- ½ teaspoon ground ginger

Instructions

1. Make the hoisin barbecue sauce by combining all of the ingredients except for the ribs in a medium bowl.

2. Trim any excess fat or flaps of meat and cut racks in half into 6- to 7-rib sections. Line a baking sheet with heavy duty aluminum foil. Place the rib racks on the baking sheet. Reserve 1 cup of the sauce and pour the rest over the rib racks. Coat both sides of racks evenly with sauce and arrange in a single layer, meaty sides up. Cover tightly with heavy duty aluminum foil and refrigerate for a minimum of four hours or overnight.

3. Preheat the oven to 300°F. Place the covered ribs in the oven and bake, undisturbed, for 1½ hours. Remove the ribs from the oven and carefully remove the foil (the steam will be very hot and can burn). Using a pastry brush or back of a spoon, coat the racks generously with the reserved barbecue sauce. Turn the oven heat up to 350 degrees. Return pan to the oven, uncovered, and cook until the ribs are tender and starting to brown, about 30 minutes. Let cool briefly before cutting in-between the ribs to serve.

4. Note: Ask your butcher to remove the white membrane on the underside of the ribs. If you need to remove it yourself, loosen it at the edge with a butter knife and peel it off (if it's slippery, grab it with a paper towel). Note that there appears to be another layer of membrane underneath the one you remove;

you shouldn't remove it as it's what holds the meat and bones together.

Prep Time: 15 Minutes

Cook Time: 30 Minutes

Servings: 12

Ingredients

- 2 cups all-purpose flour, spooned into measuring cup and leveled-off
- 2 teaspoons baking powder
- ¾ teaspoon salt
- 1 stick (½ cup) unsalted butter, softened
- 1 cup granulated sugar
- 2 large eggs
- 1½ teaspoons vanilla extract
- ¼ teaspoon almond extract
- ½ cup milk
- 2¼ cups fresh blueberries
- 2 tablespoons turbinado sugar (also called raw sugar or demerara sugar)

For Cooking:

- Non-stick cooking spray

- 12 paper muffin liners

Instructions

1. Preheat the oven to 375°F and put an oven rack in the middle position. Line a 12-cup muffin tin with paper liners. Spray the pan and the liners with non-stick cooking spray.

2. In a medium bowl, whisk together the flour, baking powder and salt.

3. In the bowl of an electric mixer, beat the butter and granulated sugar for about 2 minutes. Add the eggs one at a time, scraping down the sides of the bowl and beating well after each addition. Beat in the vanilla extract and almond extract. (The batter may look a little grainy -- that's okay).

4. Gradually add the flour mixture, alternating with the milk, beating on low speed to combine. The batter will be very thick. Add the blueberries to the batter and fold gently with a spatula until evenly distributed. Do not overmix.

5. Scoop the batter into the prepared muffin tin (an ice-cream scoop with a wire scraper works well here);

they will be very full. Sprinkle the turbinado sugar evenly on top of the muffins.

6. Bake for about 30 minutes, until lightly golden. Let the muffins cool in the pan for about 10 minutes. Run a knife around the edge of each muffin to free it from the pan if necessary (the blueberries can stick), then transfer the muffins to a rack to cool completely.

7. Freezer-Friendly Instructions: The muffins can be frozen in an airtight container or sealable plastic bag for up to 3 months. Thaw for 3 – 4 hours on the countertop before serving. To reheat, wrap individual muffins in aluminum foil and place in a preheated 350°F oven until warm.

11. French Lentil Salad with Goat Cheese

Prep Time: 15 Minutes

Cook Time: 45 Minutes

Servings: 4

Ingredients

- 1 cup French green lentils (or common brown or green lentils)
- 3 cups chicken broth
- 1 bay leaf
- 1 large carrot, finely diced
- 2 ribs celery, finely diced
- 1 teaspoon finely chopped fresh thyme (or ½ teaspoon dried)
- 3 tablespoons chopped fresh parsley
- 1 garlic clove, minced
- 1 teaspoon Dijon mustard
- 1 teaspoon honey
- ½ teaspoon salt
- ¼ teaspoon ground black pepper

- 2 tablespoons freshly squeezed lemon juice, from one lemon
- ¼ cup extra virgin olive oil, best quality such as Lucini or Colavita
- 3 ounces goat cheese

Instructions

1. Before cooking the lentils, make sure you rinse them well and pick over them to remove any small rocks or debris. Combine lentils, chicken broth and bay leaf in a medium saucepan. Bring to a boil, then turn heat down and simmer until lentils are tender, 25-30 minutes for French green lentils or 20-25 minutes for common brown or green lentils. Remove bay leaf, strain and let cool.

2. In a large bowl, combine all remaining ingredients except goat cheese. Add cooled lentils and toss to combine. Taste and adjust seasoning if necessary. Transfer salad to serving dish, crumble goat cheese over top and serve.

3. Note: When preparing this recipe, be sure to build in at least 10 minutes to cool the lentils after they have cooked.

Prep Time: 15 Minutes

Cook Time: 20 Minutes

Servings: 4

Ingredients

- 2 tablespoons extra virgin olive oil
- ¾ cup thinly sliced shallots, from 2 to 3 shallots
- 5 oz baby spinach (about 5 packed cups)
- ½ teaspoon salt
- 8 large eggs
- ⅓ cup heavy cream
- ¼ teaspoon freshly ground black pepper
- ¾ cup shredded Cheddar cheese
- ½ cup Parmigiano Reggiano
- ¼ cup fresh chopped basil

Instructions

1. Preheat the oven to 325°F, and set an oven rack in the middle position.

2. Heat the oil in a 10-inch cast iron or ovenproof nonstick skillet over medium heat. Add the shallots and cook, stirring frequently, until softened, 3 to 4 minutes. Do not brown. Add half of the spinach and cook until wilted down, about 1 minute. Add the remaining spinach and ¼ teaspoon of the salt and continue cooking until all of the spinach is wilted, 1 to 2 minutes more.

3. In a large bowl, whisk together the eggs, heavy cream, pepper, and the remaining ¼ teaspoon of salt.

4. Add the cooked spinach mixture, Cheddar, Parmigiano Reggiano, and basil to the egg mixture and stir to combine. Pour the mixture back into the pan (no need to wash it), then place it in the oven and bake until set, 20 to 23 minutes. Immediately place an oven mitt over the pan handle to remind yourself that it is hot (it's easy to forget and burn your hand, and the handle stays hot for a long time). Serve the frittata directly from the pan, or use a rubber spatula to loosen the edges and slide the frittata onto a serving platter.

5. Freezer-Friendly Instructions: The cooked frittata can be frozen for up to 3 months. Remove the frittata from the freezer about 24 hours prior to serving and reheat

it in the microwave or, covered with foil, in a 300°F oven until hot in the center.

Prep Time: 15 Minutes

Cook Time: 3hrs 20 Minutes

Servings: 15

Ingredients

Broth:

- (1) 5-6 pound whole roasting chicken (fresh or thawed)
- Salt
- Pepper
- 2 Tablespoons soft ghee (grass-fed butter, olive oil or vegan butter would work as well)
- 1 yellow onion, quartered
- 1 stalk celery, cut into 4–5 pieces
- 2 medium carrots, cut into 4 pieces each
- 1 head of garlic, cut of the top (or smash approx. 5–6 cloves)
- 1 sprig fresh rosemary
- 3–4 sprigs fresh thyme
- 1–2 fresh sage leaves

- 1 bay leaf

- 1–2 fresh sprig oregano

- 1 Tablespoon black peppercorn

Soup:

- 8 cups chicken broth (you can also use 8 cups of water to make broth completely from scratch OR you could do 4 cups broth + 4 cups water. If you use broth your soup will only turn out that much richer. Just check your ingredients on the broth if concerned with Whole30)

- Shredded chicken

- 4 stalks of celery, sliced

- 6 medium-large carrots, peeled and sliced

- 1 sweet yellow onion, diced

- 1 bay leaf

- Optional: gluten-free noodles, diced parsnip, diced sweet potato, diced turnip

Instructions

Broth:

1. Preheat oven to 375 degrees F.

2. Place chicken in 5 1/2 qt. Le Creuset Dutch Oven and rub all over with softened ghee

3. Sprinkle with generous amounts of salt and pepper to coat.

4. Place onion, carrots, celery and garlic around the chicken.

5. Roast, uncovered, for 1.5 hours.

6. Remove from oven and place on burner.

7. Add broth (and/or water) and turn heat up to high.

8. Add rosemary, thyme, sage, bay leaf, oregano and peppercorn.

9. Bring to a boil and then reduce to a simmer and cover.

10. Simmer (covered) as long as possible – if you used chicken broth I would suggest 2 hours – if you used water and broth I would suggest 3-4 hours – if you used all water I would suggest 4-6 hours.

Soup:

1. Remove chicken and set aside to cool slightly.

2. Strain broth and discard the cooked vegetables (they will be very soggy and not good for much after cooking for so long).

3. Place strained broth back in your dutch oven.

4. Once chicken is cooled enough, remove all the meat and place it in the broth (Note: depending on how big

your chicken is, feel free not use all the chicken if you feel the chicken-broth ratio is off. If you want a thicker, chunkier soup then use it all, but if you want more of a broth-based soup then reserve some of the chicken for another purpose.)

5. Also feel free to keep the chicken bones to make bone broth!

6. Once the chicken meat is back in the broth, add your onion, celery, carrots and bay leaf.

7. Taste and add salt and pepper, to taste, a pinch at a time.

8. This would also be the time to add any other ingredients you want (sweet potato, turnip, parsnip or noodles).

9. Let simmer approx. 8-10 minutes or until your vegetables are cooked, but still firm.

Notes:

1. Adaptable: This is one of those recipes that you can adapt very easily to fit what you like! My preferred method is to roast with ghee, use broth, simmer on low 2 hours (but I have also only simmered for 30 minutes – 1 hour and it is still amazing!).

2. Time Saver: Since the chicken is already fully cooked you can reduce the cooking time in Step 10 of the Broth Instructions to whatever works for you!

3. Bone Broth: you could add bone broth in Step 7 of Broth Instructions to make it extra gut-healing!

4. Noodles: If you are adding noodles I would recommend cooking them separately beforehand and then adding to the soup – otherwise as they are cooking they will soak up all of the broth.

5. Homemade Broth Version: I touched on this in the recipe card instructions, but wanted to highlight again – feel free to use water instead of broth in Instruction #7. It will need to cook much longer and you will need to add additional salt, but you will end up with some delicious homemade broth! If you have the time I highly recommend!

6. Whole30/Paleo: If you are concerned with Whole30/Paleo just check those ingredients in your broth!

Prep Time: 15 Minutes

Cook Time: 20 Minutes

Servings: 4

Ingredients

The Dressing:

- 1/2 cup mayonnaise of your choice
- 3 teaspoons dijon mustard
- 2 teaspoons garlic, minced or grated
- 1 tablespoon fresh lemon juice
- 1 teaspoon Worcestershire
- 1/4 teaspoon salt
- 1/4 teaspoon ground black pepper
- 2 teaspoons anchovy paste
- 1/2 tablespoon red wine vinegar
- 1/2 teaspoon onion powder
- 1/2 teaspoon garlic powder
- 1/4 cup parmesan cheese, grated
- The Marinade:
- 2 tablespoons olive oil (or avocado oil)

- 1 teaspoon lemon juice
- 1/4 cup soy sauce (or tamari or coconut aminos)
- 2 teaspoons worcestershire sauce
- 2 teaspoons garlic, minced
- 1/8 teaspoon kosher salt
- 1/8 teaspoon ground black pepper
- 1 teaspoon lemon zest, minced
- The Grilled Chicken Caesar Salad
- 4 medium-sized boneless, skinless chicken breasts
- 4–6 cups romaine lettuce, roughly chopped
- 2 cups croutons of your choice
- 1 cup shredded parmesan cheese

Instructions

The Dressing:

1. Combine in ingredients in a small bowl or wide mouth mason jar with lid.
2. Whisk to combine in the bowl or put the cover on your mason jar and shake to combine.
3. The Marinade:
4. Combine ingredients in a small bowl.
5. Whisk to combine.

6. Place chicken in a large dish, bowl or silicone bag. Pour over chicken and let marinate for at least 30 minutes.

7. The Grilled Chicken Caesar Salad

8. Heat grill to medium heat (approximately 400 degrees F) and ensure grill grates are clean.

9. Place chicken on direct heat (direct flame) and cook at medium heat for 4-5 minutes per side.

10. Move chicken away from the direct heat (direct flame) so that it is cooking on indirect heat (maintaining the same grill temp) and cook for an additional 5-10 minutes (you don't need to flip during this point because the chicken will cook as if it is in an oven) or until the internal temperature of the thickest part of the chicken reads 160 on your meat thermometer.

11. Remove from grill and let rest at least 5 minutes (the chicken will continue to cook during this time and the internal temp will continue to rise up to 10 additional degrees).

12. While chicken is resting divide the romaine, croutons and parmesan cheese between 4 large bowls.

13. Cut chicken into thick slices or bite-sized pieces and divide between bowls as well.

14. Serve with your favorite Homemade Caesar Dressing.

15. Enjoy!

Prep Time: 15 Minutes

Cook Time: 7hrs 20 Minutes

Servings: 14

Ingredients

- 64oz chicken stock
- 4 bone-in, skin-on chicken breasts
- 1 sweet yellow onion, chopped
- 1 bay leaf
- 1 teaspoon salt
- 1/8 teaspoon ground black pepper
- 3–4 sprigs fresh thyme
- 1 head garlic, cut off the top
- 3 medium carrots, sliced
- 4 celery stalks, sliced
- your favorite noodles

Instructions

1. Add chicken stock, chicken breasts, onion, bay leaf, salt, pepper, fresh thyme and garlic to a slow cooker.

2. Cook on LOW 8 hours or on HIGH 4 hours.

3. If cooking on HIGH: 1 hour before cooking time is done remove the chicken breasts, discard the skin and bones and shred the meat. Place back into the slow cooker along with the carrots and celery.

4. If cooking on LOW: 2 hours before cooking time is done remove the chicken breasts, discard the skin and bones and shred the meat. Place back into the slow cooker along with the carrots and celery.

5. Approximately 20 minutes before everything is done cooking, cook your favorite noodles on the stove-top until they are al dente.

6. Taste soup and add additional salt, as-needed.

7. Serve soup with noodles and enjoy!

Notes

1. Chicken Stock: you can use chicken broth if you want but chicken stock will provide more flavor.

2. Chicken Breasts: You can use boneless chicken breasts if you want, the flavor won't have quite as much depth, but then you won't have to worry about discarding the skin and bones later. Chicken thighs (boneless or bone-in) would also work!

3. Carrots + Celery: You can certainly add these right away if you want, but I personally do not like mushy

vegetables in my soup – which after slow cooking for 8 hours, the veggies will definitely be quite soft. It's up to you!

4. Noodles cooked separately: Cooking the noodles in the slow cooker can be really tricky as you have to keep in mind that as the noodles cook they are going to soak up a lot of broth in the process. Additionally, slow cookers seem to vary a lot (some run hot, some don't) so it is actually quite hard to pinpoint an exact timeframe for how long your noodles would need to cook. You can definitely cook your noodles in the slow cooker if you want, but I would suggest compensating for this by adding more broth and to watch them really closely so they don't over cook and get all mushy and gross. My preferred method is to just cook my noodles separately and then serve them together.

Prep Time: 30 Minutes

Cook Time: 20 Minutes

Servings: 6

Ingredients

- 8 Roma tomatoes; de-seeded and diced
- Approx. 30 yellow cherry tomatoes; quartered and de-seeded
- 1 tablespoon minced garlic
- 1 1/2 cup roughly chopped fresh basil leaves
- 3 tablespoons olive oil (plus some additional to brush on top of sliced baguette)
- 1 1/2 teaspoon kosher salt (more to taste)
- French baguette
- Balsamic glaze

Instructions

1. Preheat oven to 400 degrees F.
2. Combine Roma tomatoes, yellow cherry tomatoes, garlic, basil, olive oil, and salt in large mixing bowl.

3. Mix to fully combine and taste to determine if you want any additional garlic, basil or salt.

4. Let it sit for at least 30 minutes before serving.

5. Slice the french baguette at an angle to create about 1 inch thick slices.

6. Place on cookie sheet and brush with some additional olive oil.

7. Place in the oven for about 4-6 minutes, or until the bread starts to get a little crispy, watch it closely.

8. Carefully remove bread from the oven.

9. Serve slices of bread with a heaping about of the bruschetta mixture and drizzle with sweet balsamic glaze.

Prep Time: 10 Minutes

Cook Time: 05 Minutes

Servings: 4-6

Ingredients

- 2 pounds very thick asparagus, about 24 spears, ends trimmed
- 3 tablespoons extra virgin olive oil, divided
- ¼ teaspoon salt
- ¼ teaspoon freshly ground black pepper
- Zest of 1 lemon
- 1 tablespoon freshly squeezed lemon juice, from one lemon
- 3 oz feta cheese, crumbled (about ¾ cup)

Instructions

1. Preheat the grill to high.
2. Place the asparagus spears on a foil-lined baking sheet for easy clean-up. Directly on the prepared baking

sheet, toss the asparagus with 2 tablespoons of the oil, the salt and the pepper.

3. Place the asparagus spears on the grill, making sure they are perpendicular to grates so they don't fall through. Set the baking sheet near the grill (you'll need it for the cooked asparagus). Cover and cook the asparagus for 3 to 4 minutes, until nicely browned on one side and still crisp -- do not overcook. Remove the asparagus from the grill and place back on the foil-lined baking dish. Let the asparagus cool.

4. Transfer the spears to cutting board and cut on the bias into bite-sized pieces. Place the cut asparagus in a mixing bowl. Add the remaining tablespoon olive oil, lemon zest and lemon juice; toss well. Add the feta and toss gently. Taste and adjust seasoning with more salt, pepper and lemon juice (I usually add up to ¼ teaspoon more salt). Transfer to a serving platter. Serve room temperature or cold.

Prep Time: 20 Minutes

Cook Time: 15 Minutes

Servings: 2-4

Ingredients

For The Roasted Chickpeas:

- 1 (15 oz) can chickpeas, rinsed and drained
- 1 tablespoon extra virgin olive oil
- ½ teaspoon salt
- ¼ teaspoon freshly ground black pepper

For The Salad:

- 1 tablespoon freshly squeezed lemon juice, from one lemon
- 3 tablespoons extra virgin olive oil
- 1 small garlic clove, minced
- ¼ teaspoon salt
- ⅛ teaspoon freshly ground black pepper
- 1 5oz Bag or Container Baby Kale or Kale/Dark Greens Mix

- ½ cup shaved Parmigiano-Regianno

Instructions

1. Preheat oven to 425° F. Line a baking sheet with aluminum foil.
2. Place the chickpeas on the prepared baking sheet and toss with the olive oil, salt and pepper. Roast for 10-12 minutes, stirring once, until the chickpeas are slightly shrunken and crispy. Let cool.
3. In a large bowl, combine the lemon juice, olive oil, garlic, salt and pepper. Add the greens and toss until evenly coated. Taste and adjust seasoning if necessary (I usually add a bit more salt). Arrange on plates and top with Parmigiano-Regianno shavings and crispy roasted chickpeas.

Note:

1. If you can't find baby kale, feel free to substitute any other deep green blend, arugula or Lacinato kale (you'll just have to chop the leaves and let it marinate a bit).

Prep Time: 20 Minutes

Cook Time: 1hrs 15 Minutes

Servings: 6

Ingredients

Chicken:

- 4lb roasting chicken
- 3–4 tablespoons ghee, softened
- Salt and pepper
- Veggies + Potatoes
- 1 sweet yellow onion, quartered
- 3 stalks celery, cut into 1 inch chunks
- 3 medium carrots, peeled and cut in 1 inch chunks (half thicker pieces)
- 3–4 Yukon potatoes, quartered

Gravy:

- 1 tablespoon ghee
- 1 tablespoon tapioca starch
- 1 cup drippings (from bottom of Dutch Oven)
- 1/2 cup chicken broth

- salt and pepper

Instructions

2. Preheat oven to 375.
3. Place chicken in Dutch Oven.
4. Pat dry with clean paper towel.
5. Run softened ghee all over, in every nook and cranny!
6. Sprinkle generously with salt and pepper.
7. Place onion, potato, celery and carrots around chicken.
8. Place in oven, uncovered, for 1 hour and 15 minutes or until fully cooked. Use internal meat thermometer – chicken needs to reach an internal temp of 165 (at thickest part).
9. Remove from oven and let rest for 10 minutes.
10. Remove veggies and chicken from Dutch Oven and place on tray – cover with foil and set aside.
11. Take a large cast iron skillet and melt 1 tablespoon ghee. Add topioca and whisk together.
12. Slowly add the pan drippings, whisking to combine the entire time. It may get kind of chunky for a second, just keep whisking! It will smooth out and thicken.

13. Slowly add chicken broth, continuing to whisk.

14. Once gravy has thickened, taste and add salt and pepper, as desired.

15. Serve chicken, potatoes and veggies covered in gravy.

Prep Time: 10 Minutes

Cook Time: 1hrs 15 Minutes

Servings: 4-5

Ingredients

- 1 Roasted Spaghetti Squash or Instant Pot Spaghetti Squash
- 1 Tablespoon ghee or olive oil
- 1.5 lbs ground Italian sausage
- 1/2 red onion, diced (approx. 1 cup)
- 1 Tablespoon minced garlic
- Pinch of salt
- 15oz jar (approx.) of your favorite spaghetti sauce – my favorite homemade one or this one is a great option too!

Instructions

1. Ahead of time, preheat oven and roast spaghetti squash per this tutorial.

2. About 10 minutes prior to the spaghetti squash being done, take a large fry pan and olive oil (or ghee) and bring to medium-high heat.

3. Add garlic and cook for approximately 1 minute, or until fragrant, moving constantly in pan.

4. Add sausage and continue to move around pan until fully cooked.

5. Add red onion and a pinch of salt and pepper.

6. Continue cooking and stirring until onion has cooked down slightly.

7. You could add other vegetables at this point, if desired, such as mushroom or even chunks of zucchini – just add and cook for a few more minutes until cooked but firm.

8. Take medium saucepan and add your spaghetti sauce – warm on low, stirring occasionally.

9. Assemble bowl by added some spaghetti squash (top it with a chunk of ghee and a pinch of salt and pepper), a scoop or two of sausage and then as much sauce as you desire.

10. Serve immediately.

21. Roasted Eggplant Ragu + Pappardelle Noodles

Prep Time: 15 Minutes

Cook Time: 35 Minutes

Servings: 4

Ingredients

- 1 medium-sized eggplant, cut into bite-sized chunks (about 1/2 to 1 inch chunks) (make sure egpplant is fresh – older eggplant can tend to get mushy when roasted)
- 3 Tablespoons olive oil, divided
- 3–4 medium tomatoes, diced into 1 inch chunks
- 1 small yellow onion, diced
- 10 cherry tomatoes
- 1 Tablespoon red wine
- 2 Teaspoons kosher salt, divided
- 1/2 Teaspoon oregano leaves
- 1/3 Teaspoon basil leaves
- 5 garlic cloves, quartered
- 1 Teaspoon capers

- Mozzarella or burrata cheese to chunk on top.
- 1/2 cup fresh basil leaves for garnish
- Pappardelle noodles (approx. 6-9 oz) (gluten-free works too – I love this brand!)

Instructions

1. Preheat oven to 400.
2. In medium-sized bowl, add eggplant, 2 Tablespoons olive oil and 1 Teaspoon salt; toss.
3. On cookie sheet, lined with foil and sprayed with non-stick, place egpplant.
4. Roast on second from top oven rack for 20-25 minutes, stirring after 10 minutes.
5. Meanwhile, take cast iron skillet and add remaining Tablespoon of olive oil and garlic, bring to med-high heat.
6. When garlic starts to get fragrant, add onion and let cook until starts to become translucent, while stirring.
7. Then add tomatoes, wine, remaining Teaspoon of salt, oregano, basil and capers.
8. Let simmer, uncovered, for 15-20 minutes on high, or until sauce thickens – make sure to taste the sauce

and add any additional ingredients to your liking. If sauce gets too thick, add additional olive oil or wine.

9. Prepare pappardelle pasta according to packaging instructions (al dente is recommended).

10. Add eggplant and stir together.

11. Plate pappardell noodles and cover with Roasted Eggplant Ragu, chunk either mozzarella or burrata cheese (as much or as little as you like) and rip some fresh basil on top.

22. Dairy Free Dijon Chicken

Prep Time: 15 Minutes

Cook Time: 45 Minutes

Servings: 4-5

Ingredients

- 2–3 Tablespoons ghee (or olive oil)
- 1.5–2 lb boneless, skinless chicken breast OR bone-in chicken thighs
- Salt
- Pepper
- 1 can full fat coconut milk (fully incorporate with immersion blender first)
- 1 cup chicken broth
- 1/4 cup + 1 Tablespoon dijon mustard
- 1 Teaspoon fresh lemon juice
- 2 Teaspoons dried tarragon
- 1 Tablespoon arrowroot
- 10 baby Yukon gold potatoes, quartered
- Optional: 1-2 cups chopped broccolini (alternatively you can simply roast the broccolini separately and serve as a side dish) – regular broccoli work just fine

Instructions

1. Season chicken with salt and pepper.
2. In large cast iron skillet (I would recommend a 12 inch skillet/2 inches deep), heat to medium high heat and add ghee, allowing it to melt.
3. Sear chicken on each side, 3-4 minutes.
4. While chicken is cooking, combine coconut milk, chicken broth, dijon mustard, lemon juice and tarragon in medium mixing bowl; whisk to combine.
5. Pour mustard mixture around chicken and bring to simmer.
6. Let simmer, uncovered, for 10 minutes, flipping chicken halfway through.
7. Remove chicken and place on plate, setting aside.
8. Add arrowroot to pan and whisk to fully combine.
9. Add potatoes to pan and then nestle chicken.
10. Allow it to simmer for 20 minutes, uncovered, using a small whisk to continue to mix the sauce around the chicken, intermittently.
11. If adding broccolini, add with approx. 5-7 minutes left to simmer and then cover to let broccolini steam.
12. Taste and add salt, pepper or additional lemon juice, as desired.

Prep Time: 10 Minutes

Cook Time: 5 Minutes

Servings: 2

Ingredients

- 12 jumbo shrimp, deveined and shelled
- 1–2 tablespoons ghee or olive oil
- 1–2 teaspoons kosher salt
- 1/2 teaspoon ground black pepper
- 2 cups cooked brown rice
- 1 avocado, diced
- 2 tablespoons soy sauce (or tamari or coconut aminos)
- chopped cilantro (for garnish – optional)

Instructions

1. Pat shrimp dry and season with kosher salt and pepper.
2. Place large cast iron skillet on stove and bring to medium-high heat.

3. Add some of the olive oil or ghee and swirl to coat the pan.

4. Place shrimp in hot pan and let cook approx. 1-2 minutes per side or until meat is no longer translucent. Add additional oil or ghee, as needed, to keep pan from drying out.

5. Remove shrimp from pan.

6. Divide rice, avocado and shrimp between two bowls.

7. Drizzle with soy sauce (or tamari or coconut aminos) and top with a little cilantro.

8. Enjoy!

Prep Time: 10 Minutes

Cook Time: 4hrs 25 Minutes

Servings: 8-10

Ingredients

- 6–8 beef short ribs (approx. 3-4lbs)
- kosher salt and ground black pepper
- 2 tablespoons avocado or olive oil, divided
- 2 teaspoons garlic cloves, minced
- 2–3 celery stalks, sliced
- 2–3 medium carrots, peeled, sliced and quartered (halved works too)
- 1 medium sweet yellow onion, diced
- 25oz marinara sauce (homemade or store-bought)
- 1–2 bay leaves
- (optional) splash of red wine
- serving: pappardelle pasta or spaghetti squash

Instructions

1. Crock Pot / Slow Cooker

2. Place short ribs on a large plate and bring to room temperature. Pat dry with clean paper towels and season ribs with salt and pepper all over; set aside.

3. Add 1 tablespoon oil to large cast iron skillet and bring to medium-high heat.

4. Sear short ribs on all sides (do this in batches if you need to). Transfer the browned short ribs to the slow cooker.

5. In the same skillet, add another tablespoon of oil. Then add garlic and stir, allowing it to cook 1 minute.

6. Add celery, onion and carrot.

7. Sprinkle with salt and pepper.

8. Stir and allow to cook 2-3 minutes, scraping up any browned bits from the bottom of the pan.

9. Pour vegetable mixture into crockpot on top of the short ribs.

10. Pour marinara sauce on top and add bay leaves and red wine (if using). Mix to coat the short ribs.

11. Cover and let cook for 7-8 hours on low.

12. Before serving, remove short ribs and place on a plate. Shred meat using two forks, discarding bones and connective tissue. Place shredded meat back into the crockpot and mix to combine.

13. Serve with pasta, zoodles or spaghetti squash. Top
    with parmesan cheese, if desired.

Prep Time: 10 Minutes

Cook Time: 55 Minutes

Servings: 10

Ingredients

Soup:

- 1 tablespoon olive oil
- 1 tablespoon garlic, minced
- 1 small yellow onion, diced
- 6 cups chicken broth
- 1 pound boneless, skinless chicken breast
- 1 bay leaf
- 1 1/2 teaspoons kosher salt
- 1/4 teaspoon ground black pepper
- 2–3 sprigs fresh thyme
- 1–2 carrots, peeled and sliced
- 1–2 celery stalks, sliced
- 1 cup frozen peas
- 1/2 cup coconut milk
- 1/2 cup all-purpose flour

Dumpling Ingredients:

- 2 cups all-purpose flour
- 1 teaspoon kosher salt
- 1/2 cup unsweetened almond milk
- 2 eggs
- 1/2 teaspoon baking powder

Instructions

1. Bring Dutch Oven to medium-high heat. Add oil and swirl to coat the pan.
2. Add garlic and onions. Move around pan until garlic is fragrant and onions softens, about 1-2 minutes.
3. Add broth and bring to a boil. Add chicken. Cover and let chicken cook through, about 15 minutes.
4. Meanwhile, combine Dumpling Ingredients in a small bowl. Set aside.
5. Remove cooked chicken from Dutch Oven and set on a plate. Shred with two forks. Set aside.
6. Ensure broth is very hot and then using a glass measuring cup with a handle, carefully scoop out two cups of hot broth. Add in 1/2 cup flour and whisk immediately.

7. Add the broth/flour mixture back into the Dutch Oven. Stir to combine.

8. Add in the shredded chicken, bay leaf, kosher salt, ground black pepper, thyme, carrots, celery and coconut milk.

9. Bring to a simmer and stir fairly constantly as it thickens, about 5-8 minutes.

10. Take your dumpling dough and add to soup 1/2 tablespoon at a time. Once all the dumpling dough has been used cover the Dutch Oven and let gently simmer 5-10 minutes or until dumplings are fully cooked.

11. Add the frozen peas and mix to fully combine. Cover and remove from heat. Let stand 5-10 minutes or until peas are fully thawed.

12. Serve immediately.

Prep Time: 10 Minutes

Cook Time: 40 Minutes

Servings: 8

Ingredients

- 1 tablespoon olive oil
- 1 tablespoon garlic, minced
- 1 small yellow onion, diced
- 1 medium carrot, chopped
- 1 celery stalk, chopped
- 6 cups chicken broth
- 1 pound boneless, skinless chicken breasts
- 1/4 cup all-purpose flour
- 6oz tomato paste
- 1 cup full fat coconut milk
- 1/2 tablespoon coconut sugar
- 1 teaspoon kosher salt
- 1/8 teaspoon ground black pepper
- 1 teaspoon Italian seasoning
- Approx. 9oz tortellini (I used Kite Hill dairy-free tortellini)

- (optional) handful chopped kale or spinach

Instructions

1. Bring Dutch Oven to medium-high heat. Add oil; swirl to coat the pan.
2. Add garlic and onion. Move around pan until garlic is fragrant and onions soften, about 1 minute.
3. Add carrots and celery and saute for 1-2 minutes.
4. Add chicken broth and bring to a boil. Add chicken breasts. Cover and let simmer until fully cooked, about 15 minutes.
5. Remove chicken and place on a plate to cool a bit.
6. Carefully remove 1 cup of very hot broth (we recommend using a measuring cup with a handle) from the pot. Add flour and whisk immediately until it thickens. Return mixture to Dutch Oven. Stir until soup thickens.
7. Add tomato paste and coconut milk. Stir to combine. Bring to a simmer as mixture continues to thicken.
8. Shred chicken with two forks and return meat to pot along with coconut sugar, salt, pepper, Italian seasoning and tortellini. Let simmer approx. 10-15

minutes or until tortellini is fully cooked. Taste and adjust any seasoning, as desired.

9. If using, add in a handful of chopped kale or spinach right before serving.

Prep Time: 20 Minutes

Cook Time: 35 Minutes

Servings: 6

Ingredients

Whipped Feta:

- 8oz feta cheese
- 1 cup plain greek yogurt
- 4 teaspoons high-quality olive oil
- 2 teaspoon finely grated lemon zest
- 1 teaspoon fresh mint leaves, minced
- 2 teaspoon garlic, minced
- 1/4 teaspoon salt
- 1/8 teaspoon ground black pepper

Lemon Garlic Quinoa:

- 1 tablespoon olive oil
- 2 teaspoons garlic, minced
- 2 1/4 cups water or chicken broth
- 1 1/4 cups quinoa
- 2–3 teaspoon lemon zest

- 2 tablespoon lemon juice

- 1 teaspoon kosher salt

- 1/2 teaspoon dried oregano leaves

- 1/4 teaspoon dried thyme leaves

Greek Meatballs:

- 1 pound ground lamb

- 1 egg

- 1/2 cup fine almond flour

- 1 teaspoon salt

- 1 teaspoon dried oregano leaves

- 1 teaspoon dried basil

- 1 teaspoon dried dill

- 1/2 teaspoon onion powder

- 1 teaspoon garlic powder

- 1/2 teaspoon ground black pepper

- 1 tablespoon fresh mint, minced

- 1 teaspoon garlic, minced

Instructions

Whipped Feta:

1. Add ingredients to food processor (crumble the feta so it whips more easily).
2. Process mixture on high until the consistency is smooth.
3. Taste and adjust any salt or other flavor, as necessary.
4. Lemon Garlic Quinoa:
5. Bring a medium saucepan to medium-high heat. Add oil and swirl to coat the pan. Add garlic and move around the pan until fragrant, about 30 seconds.
6. Add water (or chicken broth), quinoa, lemon juice and salt. Stir to combine.
7. Bring to boil then reduce to a simmer and let cook 8-10 minutes or until the water has been absorbed.
8. Add lemon zest, oregano and thyme. Stir to combine. Taste and add any additional lemon zest, salt or herbs – as desired.

Greek Meatballs:

1. Combine ingredients in a medium mixing bowl; mix.
2. Taking one tablespoon of lamb mixture at a time, create meatballs with your hand or a small dough scoop. Place on a plate.
3. Bring large cast iron skillet to medium-high heat. Add approximately a tablespoon of olive oil to the pan; swirl to coat.

4. Sear the meatballs on all sides.

5. Turn heat down to medium/medium-low and continue cooking unit internal temperature reaches 145 degrees F (about 10-15 minutes).

Serving:

1. Divide Lemon Garlic Quinoa, Whipped Feta and Greek meatballs between bowls. Garnish with some Quick Pickled Veggies if you want!

Prep Time: 15 Minutes

Cook Time: 35 Minutes

Servings: 15

Ingredients

- 1 tablespoon olive oil
- 1 tablespoon garlic, minced
- 1/2 cup yellow onion, diced
- 4 heaping cups shredded chicken
- 8oz can green chiles
- 1 teaspoon kosher salt
- 1/4 teaspoon ground black pepper
- 1 teaspoon garlic powder
- 1/2 teaspoon cumin
- Approx. 2 cups enchilada sauce
- 12 regular size tortillas, cut in half (flour or corn)
- 15oz can refried beans (black beans work too)
- Approx. 3 cups shredded cheese of your choice

Instructions

1. Preheat oven to 350 degrees F.

2. Bring a large cast iron skillet to medium-high heat.

3. Add oil; swirl to coat the pan.

4. Add garlic and move around pan until fragrant, approx. 30 seconds.

5. Add onion and move around pan until it softens slightly, approx. 1 minute.

6. Add chicken, green chiles, salt, pepper, garlic powder and cumin. Stir until combined and chicken is warmed through.

7. Take a 9×13 baking pan and add about a tablespoon or so of sauce on the bottom.

8. Top with a layer of tortillas (cut them in half and place the cut sides along the edge of the pan – two on each long side and one on each short side with one covering the middle).

9. Continue layering by adding 1/2 the beans, 1/2 the chicken mixture, approx. 1/2 cup enchilada sauce and then 1/3 cup cheese.

10. Repeat layers: tortillas, beans, chicken, sauce, cheese.

11. End with another layer of tortillas, the remaining sauce and then the remaining cheese.

12. Spray a piece of foil with olive oil or your favorite non-stick and cover the pan (non-stick side down) and place in the oven, middle rack, for 30 minutes.

13. Remove foil and return to oven for 5-10 minutes or until cheese is melted and sauce is a bit bubbly.

14. Remove and let cool slightly before serving.

15. We love serving this with some sour cream, fresh cilantro and some Salsa Rice!

Prep Time: 15 Minutes

Cook Time: 25 Minutes

Servings: 2

Ingredients

Chicken:

- 1 boneless, skinless chicken breast
- 1 batch chipotle seasoning

Salad:

- 4 cups romaine or mixed greens
- 1 cup black beans, drained and rinsed
- 1/4 cup green onion, sliced
- 1/2 cup corn (canned or grilled)
- 1 red bell pepper, diced
- 1 cup cherry tomatoes, halved
- 1/2 cup cotija cheese, crumbled
- 1/4 cup black olives, sliced
- 1/2 cup corn chips, crushed
- (optional) 2-4 jalapeno sliced

- toppings: guacamole, pico de gallo/salsa and sour cream
- Dressing: creamy southwest dressing or southwest vinaigrette

Instructions

Chicken:

1. Combine chipotle seasoning in small bowl; stir to combine (Note: if you don't want to use chipotle seasoning feel free to use any seasoning you want or you can just use kosher salt and ground black pepper).
2. Place chicken breasts on plate and pat dry.
3. Sprinkle all over with chipotle seasoning and rub all over.
4. Drizzle with olive oil and fully coat.
5. Heat grill to medium heat (approximately 400 degrees).
6. Place chicken on direct heat (direct flame) and cook at medium heat for 4-5 minutes per side.
7. Move chicken away from the direct heat (direct flame) so that it is cooking on indirect heat (maintaining the same grill temp) and cook for an additional 7-10 minutes (you don't need to flip during this point

because the chicken will cook as if it is in an oven) or until the internal temperature of the thickest part of the chicken reads 160 on your meat thermometer.

8. Remove from grill and let rest at least 5 minutes (the chicken will continue to cook during this time and the internal temp will continue to rise up to 10 additional degrees). Chicken is safe to eat when it reaches an internal temp of 165 degrees (at thickest part of the breast).

9. Slice or cube the chicken.

Salad:

1. Divided ingredients between two bowls.
2. Use the toppings of your choice
3. Top with your choice of Creamy Southwest Dressing or Southwest Vinaigrette.

Prep Time: 15 Minutes

Cook Time: 25 Minutes

Servings: 20-24

Ingredients

- Chicken Meatballs:
- 1lb ground chicken
- 1 large egg
- 1/2 cup Bob's Red Mill Almond Flour
- 1 teaspoon onion powder
- 1/2 teaspoon garlic powder
- 1 teaspoon salt
- 1/2 teaspoon ground black pepper

Tikka Masala Sauce:

- 1–2 tablespoon ghee
- 1 sweet yellow onion, diced
- 2 teaspoon fresh ginger, grated
- 1–2 tablespoons garlic, minced
- 1/2 teaspoon ground turmeric
- 2 teaspoons ground coriander

- 2 teaspoons ground paprika
- 1/2 teaspoon ground cumin
- 1–2 teaspoons garam masala
- 1/4 teaspoon red chili powder
- 15oz can tomato sauce
- 1 teaspoon fresh lemon juice
- 1 cup full fat coconut milk

Topping:

- Fresh cilantro, chopped

Instructions

1. Bring a medium saucepan to medium-high heat and add ghee. Once ghee has melted, add garlic. Let cook, moving around the pan, until aromatic, about 1 minute. Add onions and let cook down, about 2-3 minutes.

2. Add ginger, garlic, turmeric, coriander, paprika, cumin, garam masala and red chili powder. Stir to combine.

3. Pour in tomato sauce, lemon juice and coconut milk. Stir to combine and bring to just under a simmer. Cover.

4. To make the chicken meatballs, combine ground chicken, egg, almond flour, onion powder, garlic powder, salt and black pepper in a medium mixing bowl.

5. Use a cookie dough scoop to scoop out approx. 1 1/2 tablespoons of meatball mixture, forming a ball, and place on a large plate. Continue until all of the meatball mixture is used. (See Notes)

6. Take large/medium cast iron skillet and bring to medium-high heat. Add a tablespoon of oil and use a spatula to spread evenly to coat the pan. Add chicken meatballs and sear on all sides, about 3 minutes.

7. Turn down heat to medium and then add the tikka masala sauce. Cover and let simmer 15 minutes, stirring occasionally. Use a meat thermometer to ensure meatballs have reached in internal temp of 165 to ensure they are fully cooked.

8. Serve with cauliflower rice (Whole30/Paleo) or with regular rice and top with fresh cilantro.

www.ingramcontent.com/pod-product-compliance
Lightning Source LLC
Chambersburg PA
CBHW051832250726
48659CB00005B/1801